Copyright 2023

Table of Contents

PREVIEW

IVF helps people with infertility who want to have a baby. Because it's expensive and invasive, couples often try other fertility treatments first. These may include taking fertility drugs or having intrauterine insemination.

IVF or in vitro fertilisation is a series of procedures to assist you with conception. It is when a human egg is fertilised with sperm in a laboratory. If the fertilised egg (embryo) successfully implants in the uterus, this will result in pregnancy.

In Vitro Fertilization is an assisted reproductive technology (ART) commonly referred to as IVF. IVF is the process of fertilization by extracting eggs, retrieving a sperm sample, and then manually combining an egg and sperm in a laboratory dish. The embryo(s) is then transferred to the uterus. Other forms of ART include gamete intrafallopian transfer (GIFT) and zygote intrafallopian transfer (ZIFT).

In vitro fertilization, known as IVF, is a procedure used to help you get pregnant.

In IVF, a human egg is fertilised with sperm in a laboratory then implanted into a uterus. If the fertilised egg (embryo) successfully implants in the uterus, this will result in pregnancy.

IVF may be used to treat infertility, to prevent certain genetic problems or to help people who are single or in the sexually- and gender-diverse (LGBTIAQ+) community start a family.

IVF success rates vary — your doctor can help you understand your chances of becoming pregnant with IVF.

IVF can be expensive, so it's a good idea to discuss the pros and cons of fertility treatment with your treatment provider and your partner (if you have one) before you start.

IN VITRO FERTILIZATION DIET RECIPES

BREAKFAST

1. Sausage Egg Bake Casserole

Prep Time: 10 Minutes

Cook Time: 40 Minutes

Servings: 6

Ingredients

- 5 sausages (your favorite kind)
- 6 strips bacon
- 7 oz spinach leaves (200g)
- 1 bell pepper (red, orange or yellow)
- 4 scallions (spring onions green onions)
- 3.3 oz shredded cheddar (100g)
- 5 oz cherry tomatoes (150g)

For the egg mix

- 12 large free range eggs
- 3.5 oz milk (100ml)
- ¼ teaspoon black pepper
- 2 tablespoons dried mixed herbs

- .125 tsp salt (to taste)

Instructions

Cook the meats

- Preheat the oven to 390°f 200°c and line a baking tray with foil.
- Place the sausages and bacon on the tray and cook for around 20 minutes until done. Remove from the oven and let cool. KEEP THE OVEN ON!
- When cool enough, slice the sausage in to bite sized pieces and break up the bacon.

Make the egg mix

1. Mix all of the ingredients for the egg mix together in a large jug and set aside
2. Prep the veggies
3. Dice the bell pepper and clean and slice the scallions. Half the cherry tomatoes.
4. Build the casserole
5. In an oven proof dish, spread out half of the spinach across the bottom, then evenly distribute half of the bell pepper, two scallions, half of the sausage and bacon and sprinkle over half of the cheese.

6. Repeat to use up the rest of the ingredients; a layer of spinach then the bell pepper, scallions, sausage and bacon. Don't add the cheese yet! Add the cherry tomato halves instead.

7. Pour over the egg mix and then sprinkle over the remaining cheese.

8. Bake the casserole

9. Place the casserole into the pre heated oven (390°f 200°c) for around 40 minutes. keep an eye on it - you can pop a bit of foil over the top if it's getting a bit too dark! Use a knife to check that the egg is cooked through, if you have an instant read thermometer, the bake should be 160°f 71°c.

2. Air Fryer Lamb Meatballs

Prep Time: 10 Minutes

Cook Time: 15 Minutes

Servings: 12

Ingredients

- 1 pound ground lamb (510g)
- ¼ teaspoon salt
- ¼ teaspoon black pepper
- ½ teaspoon garlic powder
- ½ teaspoon onion powder
- 3 tablespoons fine breadcrumbs
- ¼ cup fresh parsley (chopped)
- oil

Instructions

1. Preheat the air fryer to 380F / 190c.
2. Add all of the ingredinets, except the oil, to a large bowl, and combine using your hands.
3. Roll the mixture into balls, about two tablespoons each, and place on a lined baking sheet til ready to cook.

4. Spray the air fryer basket with oil to coat it and place in the meatballs in an even layer. Spray the tops of the meatballs with more oil.
5. Set to cook at 380F / 190c for 15 minutes, shake halfway through cooking.
6. Add to hot pasta sauce and serve over freshly cooked

3. Twice Baked Potatoes Recipe

Prep Time: 20 Minutes

Cook Time: 1hr 50 Minutes

Servings: 4

Ingredients

- 2 baking potatoes
- 4 pork sausages
- 5.3 ounces mushrooms finely chopped (150g)
- 2 eggs
- 3.5 ounces cream cheese (100g)
- 3.5 ounces strong grated cheddar (100g)
- 4 spring onions (scallions) finely sliced
- 3 tbsp wholegrain mustard
- salt and pepper

Instructions

1. Pre-heat the oven to 430f 220°c. Rub the potatoes in a little oil, sprinkle with salt and put in the oven for 1 - 1 ½ hours until crispy on the outside. Leave to one side to cool. Keep the oven at 220°.

2. In a frying pan, cook the sausages through. Leave to one side. In the same pan, fry the mushrooms for about 10 minutes until golden brown.

3. Cut the potatoes lengthways, and scoop out the insides into a large bowl. You want to leave a thin layer of potato on the skins so they keep their shape. To the flesh, add the eggs and cream cheese, beat together well with a fork until you get a creamy consistency.

4. Cut the sausages into small chunks and add to the bowl along with the mushrooms, cheddar, onions, mustard and chilli. Give it another good mix and add a few good pinches of salt and pepper to season.

5. Spoon the mixture back into the potato skins - fill them right up! Then wrap two pieces of bacon around each potato half. Put back in the oven at 430f 220°c for around 30mins until the bacon is crispy.

4. Air Fryer Sausage and Egg Breakfast Casserole

Prep Time: 5 Minutes

Cook Time: 40 Minutes

Servings: 4

Ingredients

- ½ green bell pepper (diced)
- 1 small onion (diced)
- 3 pork breakfast sausages (sliced into bite sized picces)
- ¼ cup shredded mozzarella (4 tablespoons)

For the egg mix

- 6 eggs
- ¼ cup cream (35%) (4 tablespoons)
- ¼ teaspoon salt
- pinch black pepper
- ½ teaspoon garlic powder

Instructions

1. Preheat the air fryer to 400F.

2. Place the diced bell pepper and onion into a baking dish and add in the sliced sausage.

3. Cook at 400F for 10 minutes, stirring halfway through, til the sausage is browned and the veggies are soft.

4. While that is cooking, mix together the ingredients for the egg mix in a jug (eggs, cream, salt, pepper and garlic powder).

5. Once the sausage and veggies are cooked, top with the shredded cheese and pour the egg mix over the top.

6. Cook at 260F for 30 to 35 minutes til the egg is cooked all the way through.

5. Breakfast Stuffed Peppers

Prep Time: 10 Minutes

Cook Time: 40 Minutes

Servings: 4

Ingredients

- 2 large bell peppers (your colour of choice!)
- 1 cooked sausage
- ½ jalapeno pepper finely dliced
- 12 cherry tomatoes halved
- ¾ ounce Shredded cheddar cheese (divided) (25g)
- 3 eggs
- ⅓ cup milk or heavy cream (80ml)
- salt and pepper (to taste)
- 1 tbsp chives (optional, to serve) finely chopped

Instructions

1. Pre heat the oven to 180°c 350°f
2. Cut the peppers in half through the stalk and scoop out the seeds and any white pith.

3. Divide the cooked sausage, jalapeno, cherry tomatoes and half the cheese between each pepper half.

4. Mix the eggs with the milk and a little salt and pepper. Pour this into the pepper halves (not right to the top or they will overflow when cooked).

5. Sprinkle the top of each pepper with the remainder of the cheese.

6. Put the pepper halves on a baking tray and put in the pre heated oven for 40 minutes until the egg has turned solid.

6. Fried Bread English Sandwich

Prep Time: 5 Minutes

Cook Time: 25 Minutes

Servings: 2

Ingredients

- 2 pork sausages
- 1 avocado
- ½ tspn English mustard
- ½ tspn Worcestershire sauce
- 2 strips bacon
- 1 plum tomato
- 4 slices tiger bread
- 3.5 ounces salted butter (100g)
- paprika
- 2 eggs
- mayonaise
- salt and pepper
- olive oil

Instructions

1. Heat the oven to 200° and pop the sausages in for 25mins. Whilst they are cooking you can prep the rest.

2. Mash the avocado in a bowl, and add in the english mustard, worcestershire sauce and a sprinkling of salt and pepper. Combine well and leave to one side.

3. In a large frying pan and fry the bacon, no need to add any oil in (I really do recommend you use the American streaky kind so you get a real crunch!). Keep the frying pan hot and place the bacon to one side. Slice the tomato as thinly as you and put the slices into the hot frying pan and fry for about 3-4 minutes on each side, until they are slightly coloured and soft. Scoop out of the pan and leave to one side.

4. To the hot pan, add in 50g of butter and that will start to foam. Add in the slices of bread and sprinkle a little salt, pepper and paprika on the top whilst the underside fries. Whilst it is frying move the pan around so that the bread is allowed to soak up all the butter. When golden and crispy on one side, flip the slices, this should take about 4-5mins. Add in cubes of the remaining butter and fry to perfection. Once cooked, leave to one side.

5. Rinse out the pan and over a medium high flame heat a good amount of oil - you want enough to cover the

base of the whole pan. To fry the eggs, I used a couple of chefs rings to keep a really nice shape. Pop the rings onto the hot oil and break and egg into each. Spoon hot oil over the top, and carefully remove once cooked.

6. The sausages should be cooked by now, so remove these from the oven. Now to stack!

7. For each sandwich, dollop a thin layer of mayonnaise on top of two slices of the fried bread, then spoon over a generous helping of the avocado mixture. Cut a sausage in half lengthways and place on top of the sausage. Spoon over half of the tomatoes, top with a couple of strips of bacon and then the fried egg on top. Place the other slice of fried bread and avocado on top.

7. Bison Meatballs

Prep Time: 10 Minutes

Cook Time: 15 Minutes

Servings: 12

Ingredients

- 21 ounces ground bison (600g)
- ¼ cup fine breadcrumbs (4 tablespoons)
- 1 tablespoon Italian seasoning
- ½ teaspoon salt
- ½ teaspoon black pepper
- 1 egg
- 1 tablespoon Worcestershire sauce
- oil for frying

Instructions

1. Add all of the ingredients to a large bowl (apart from the oil).
2. Mix the ingredients together using your hands so that everything is well incorporated.

3. Take portions of the mixture and roll into balls. I used around 3 tablespoons per meatball. Place on a tin lined with parchment.

To pan fry

1. Add a tablespoon of oil to a large skillet and heat on a medium high heat.
2. Once hot, add the meatballs, taking care not to overcrowd the pan. Cook on all sides until browned and cooked through - about 10-15 minutes.

To oven bake

1. Pre heat the oven to 400F 200c.
2. Place the meatballs into the oven on a baking sheet lined with parchment and cook for 20-25 minutes until browned and cooked through.

8. Air Fryer Bacon Wrapped Hot Dogs

Prep Time: 5 Minutes

Cook Time: 10 Minutes

Servings: 4

Ingredients

- 4 hot dogs
- 4 strips bacon
- To serve
- hot dog buns
- mustard, ketchup and any other toppings you enjoy.

Instructions

1. Soak the toothpicks in cold water if using.
2. Preheat the air fryer to 380F 190c.
3. Wrap each hot dog with a strip of bacon, securing both ends with a toothpick.
4. Once the air fryer is preheated, place the hot dogs n the basket in a single layer and set to cook at 380F 190c for 10 minutes.

5. Turn the hot dogs carefully halfway through cooking so that they cook evenly.

6. Cook til the bacon is done to your liking (for me it was 10 minutes) and serve in buns with your favorite toppings.

9. Air Fryer Sausage Peppers Onions and Potatoes

Prep Time: 5 Minutes

Cook Time: 25 Minutes

Servings: 3

Ingredients

For the potatoes

- 1 pound red potatoes
- 1 tablespoon oil
- ½ teaspoon paprika
- ½ teaspoon garlic powder
- ¼ teaspoon salt
- pinch black pepper

For the sausages and veggies

- 1 Spanish onion
- 1 red bell pepper
- 6 Italian sausages
- 1 tablespoon oil
- ½ teaspoon paprika
- ½ teaspoon garlic powder
- ¼ teaspoon salt

- pinch black pepper

Instructions

1. Preheat the air fryer to 400F / 200c.
2. Wash the potatoes and chop into bitesized pieces.
3. Place the potatoes into a large bowl and add the oil and seasonings. Mix well so that the potato chunks are coated.
4. Add the potatoes into the air fryer and set to cook at 400f 200c for 5 minutes.
5. Meanwhile, peel and slice the onion, cut the bell pepper into chunks and slice the sausages into bitesized pieces. Place in the bowl the potatoes were in, add the oil and seasonings and mix well.
6. Once the potatoes have cooked for 5 minutes, add the seasoned sausages and veggies to the air fryer basket.
7. Set to cook at 370F 190c for 20 minutes.
8. Stir the ingredients in the basket around every 5 to 7 minutes to help cook evenly.
9. Serve!

10. Egg White Frittata

Prep Time: 10 Minutes

Cook Time: 30 Minutes

Servings: 4

Ingredients

- 2 cups egg whites (16 egg whites 17.5fl oz 500ml)
- ½ cup heavy cream (36%) (100ml)
- 1 tablespoon dried oregano
- ¼ teaspoon salt
- ¼ teaspoon pepper
- 1 tablespoon oil (for cooking)
- 1 red bell pepper (sliced)
- 1 red onion (sliced)
- 2 garlic cloves (minced)
- 2 handfuls spinach leaves

Instructions

1. Pre heat the oven to 400F 200c.
2. Whisk together the egg whites, cream, oregano, salt and pepper and set to one side.

3. Heat the oil in a skillet on a medium high heat. Once hot add the sliced onion and pepper with a pinch of salt and pepper and cook until soft.

4. Add in the garlic and cook for an extra minute.

5. Add in the spinach and stir it in to wilt it.

6. Pour the egg white mix into the skillet.

7. Move the skillet into the oven and bake for 15 to 20 minutes until the egg has set.

8. Let cool for 5 minutes before slicing and serving.

LUNCH

11. Steak Tartare

Prep Time: 30 Minutes

Cook Time: 00 Minutes

Servings: 4

Ingredients

For the steak tartare

- 2 sirloin steaks (around 7 ounces 200g each)
- 1 tbsp Worcestershire sauce
- 1 tbsp red wine vinegar
- ½ tbsp dijon mustard
- ounces chives finely chopped (10g)

For the pickled shallots

- ounces shallots - 2 or 3 (100g)
- 5 ounces red wine vinegar (150ml)
- salt and pepper
- 1 tbsp sugar

To Serve

- 2 ounces capers (50g)

- 8-10 cornichons
- 2-4 slices of toasted bread
- 4 egg yolks

Instructions

1. First off, put your steaks in the freezer, this will make them easier to dice.

2. Finely slice the shallots and place into a small saucepan with the red wine vinegar, a pinch of salt and pepper and the caster sugar. Bring to the boil and then let simmer. Keep cooking until all of the liquid has evaporated. Take off the heat and let cool.

3. Take one steak out of the freezer. as thin as you can, slice the steak in to strips, discarding any fat or sinew. Slice each strip, again, as thin as you can, and then dice these strips. Repeat with the other steak.

4. Put the steak pieces into a bowl and add the Worcester sauce, red wine vinegar, mustard, gin, chives and a good couple of pinches of salt and pepper. Mix well. Taste a piece of steak to check the seasoning and add more salt and pepper if needed. Place into the fridge until ready to plate up - don't leave for more than 30mins.

5. Roughly chop the capers.

6. Use a chefs ring, or cookie cutter to place the steak tartare on to the plates. Don't compact the steak down. Using a teaspoon, make a small dip in the middle of the meat and carefully place in an egg yolk. Remove the

ring and place the capers, onions and cornichons around the steak, along with the toast.

7. Serve immediately.

12. Oven Baked Red Pesto Frittata

Prep Time: 5 Minutes

Cook Time: 25 Minutes

Servings: 4

Ingredients

- 6 eggs
- 3 tablespoons sour cream
- 3 tablespoons red pesto
- 1 tablespoon Italian seasoning
- 1 teaspoon oil
- 2 garlic cloves minced
- 1 red onion sliced
- 1 red bell pepper diced
- 12 to 16 cherry tomatoes halved
- 12 asparagus stems cut into quarters
- salt and pepper to taste

Instructions

1. Pre heat the oven to 360F 180c

2. In a jug, whisk together the eggs, sour cream, pesto and Italian seasoning. Set to one side.

3. Heat the oil in a large skillet or frying pan on a medium heat.

4. Add the garlic and onion and cook until it starts to soften.

5. Add in the bell pepper, cherry tomatoes and asparagus with a pinch of salt and pepper. Cook until the veggies are softened, about 5 to 10 minutes.

6. Pour over the egg mixture and cook until the bottom starts to solidify but the top is still runny.

7. Move the skillet into the oven and bake for 10 to 15 minutes until the egg is cooked through and the top is browned.

8. Let sit for 5 to 10 minutes before serving.

13. Buffalo Chicken Lettuce Wraps

Prep Time: 5 Minutes

Cook Time: 10 Minutes

Servings: 4

Ingredients

- 3 cups cooked shredded chicken (300g)
- ¾ cup buffalo sauce (175ml)
- 3 tablespoons salted butter
- romain or bibb lettuce leaves
- blue cheese
- ranch dressing

Instructions

1. Place the shredded chicken in a pot with the buffalo sauce and butter.
2. Heat on on a medium high heat, stirring occasionally to combine. Cook for 5 to 10 minutes until the chicken is heated through.

3. Place a couple of tablespoons of the chicken on to lettuce leaves, top with blue cheese crumbles and a drizzle of ranch dressing.
4. Serve immediately.

14. Beetroot & Gorgonzola Tart

Prep Time: 20 Minutes

Cook Time: 1hr 30 Minutes

Servings: 8

Ingredients

- 6 sheets of ready made filo pastry
- 1 beaten egg
- 1 ounce walnuts crushed in a mortar and pestle (25g)
- 3 beetroots
- 4 tbsp sugar
- 3 red onions finely sliced
- 4 ounces balsamic vinegar (100ml)
- 1.75 ounces red wine vinegar (50ml)
- 1.75 ounces olive oil (50ml)
- 3 eggs
- 10 ounces creme fraiche (300ml)
- 2 tbsp fresh chives finely chopped
- 7 ounces gorgonzola (200g)

Instructions

1. Pre-heat the oven to 390f 200°c.

2. Peel and top and tail the beetroots and cut them into ½ cm slices. Put on a roasting tray and sprinkle with a table spoon of caster sugar and a good pinch of salt. Place in the oven for about 20mins. Test with a knife - they should be soft with little resistance, and put to one side to cool.

3. Put the sliced onions into a saucepan and add the balsamic and red wine vinegar, along with the olive oil and 3 tablespoons of caster sugar. Put on a medium heat and stir occasionally until the liquid has evaporated. This should take about 30 minutes. Leave to one side to cool.

4. Lightly grease the dish you will be baking the tart in.

5. Take a sheet of filo and place it your dish so that the pastry comes up the sides slightly (fold the edges over if needed). Gently brush with some beaten egg and sprinkle over a small amount of the crushed walnuts. Lay another piece of filo over the top and repeat the process until you have placed on your last layer of filo. Brush well with the beaten egg and put in the oven for 10mins. Once golden brown, leave to one side to cool.

6. Turn the oven down to 355°f 180°c.

7. In a bowl, whisk together the eggs, creme fraiche and chives. Add salt and pepper to taste. Cut the gorgonzola into small cubes and stir in to the egg and cream.

8. Take the filo case, and evenly spread over the onion mixture. Place the roasted beetroot slices on top and then pour over the egg and cream mixture. Pop in the oven for 40mins, until the filling has set and the top is golden brown. Let cool before serving.

15. Slow Roasted Chicken with Garlic, Lemon and Herbs

Prep Time: 30 Minutes

Cook Time: 3hrs 2 Minutes

Servings: 5

Ingredients

- 1 whole chicken about 2.6 pounds (1.2kg)
- Juice and zest of 2 lemons
- 2 whole lemons
- 1 garlic bulb
- 1 large bunch of fresh thyme
- 1 bunch of sage
- ounces salted butter (150g)
- Salt & pepper

Instructions

1. Let the chicken get up to room temp before you start and gently pat off any excess moisture with kitchen paper. Pre heat the oven to 300F 150°c.
2. In a bowl, mix 50g of softened butter with the zest of two lemons, 1 garlic clove and the leaves from a couple

of sprigs of thyme and 3-4 chopped sage leaves. Leave to one side.

3. Put a couple of good pinches of salt and cracked black pepper into the cavity of the chicken. Take a lemon and stab it a few times with a fork. Pop the lemon, most of the sage, 8 sprigs of time and 4 garlic cloves (the cloves don't need to be pealed, just lightly bashed) into the cavity.

4. Using a spoon, gently lift the skin away from the breasts. Be careful you don't pierce the skin. Take the butter mixture and spoon this between the gap you have created between the skin and the breast. use your hands to push this as far down the chicken as you can. Spread any left over butter mixture of the top of the chicken.

5. In a small pan melt 100g of butter and mix with the juice of two lemons, 1 chopped garlic clove and leaves from a couple of sprigs of thyme and a couple of chopped sage leaves. Once it is all mixed and melted, use the syringe to inject this mixture into the chicken meat. Use about half. YOU CAN SKIP THIS STEP IF YOU DON'T HAVE A MEAT INJECTOR

6. Place the chicken, breast side down in a roasting tin, and pop any left over herbs around it, along with slices

of lemon and the rest of the garlic cloves. Cover loosely with tin foil and put in the oven.

7. Roast the covered chicken for 2 hours.

8. Just before the two hours is up, heat the leftover butter mixture that you used to inject the chicken.

9. Remove the chicken from the oven and discard the foil. Carefully turn over the chicken so it is breast side up and pour over the melted butter mixture. Place back in the oven for another hour.

10. To check it's ready, use a meat thermometer which should register at 165F, or check the juices run clear when you pierce the skin.

11. For a super crispy brown skin, place the chicken under the broiler (grill) on medium/high for 5 to 10 minutes, watching closely so it doesn't burn.

12. Let the chicken sit for 15-20mins, covered, before carving and serving.

16. Grilled Lemon and Herb Chicken Salad

Prep Time: 10 Minutes

Cook Time: 15 Minutes

Servings: 4

Ingredients

For the marinated chicken

- 2 chicken breast (organic and free range)
- 2 tbsp olive oil
- ½ tbsp dried oregano
- ½ tbsp dried basil
- ½ tbsp dried rosemary
- ¼ tbsp ground black pepper
- ⅛ tsp salt
- ¼ tsp garlic powder
- juice and zest of 2 lemons

For the salad

- ½ iceberg or romaine lettuce shredded
- ½ small red onion finely sliced
- 1 red pepper finely sliced
- ½ cucumber finely sliced

- 12 cherry tomatoes cut in half
- 1 avocado sliced
    - to 5 ounces marinated feta cheese (100 to 150g)
- 2 sundried tomatoes finely sliced
- 1 tbsp sesame seeds
- ground black pepper
- For the salad dressing
- ¾ cup extra virgin olive oil
- ¼ cup white wine vinegar
- 1 garlic clove minced
- 1 tbsp Italian seasoning
- ¼ tsp ground black pepper
- juice and zest of ½ lemon
- ¼ tsp salt
- 1 tbsp sugar

Instructions

To marinade the chicken

1. Put all of the ingredients for the marinaded chicken (except for the chicken) into a jug and mix well.
2. Put the chicken breasts into a zip lock bag, and pour over the marinade. Close the bag and use your hands to

move the marinade around and coat the chicken. Put in the fridge for at least 30 mins - up to 2 hours for a stronger flavor.

3. For the salad dressing

4. Mix together all of the ingredients for the dressing and store in the fridge until ready to use.

To put it all together

1. When you are ready to cook the chicken, add a little oil to a grill pan and put on a medium high heat. Cook on both sides for around 15 to 20 minutes til cooked through. You can also use an outdoor grill.

2. While the chicken is cooking you can prep the salad. Layer the iceberg lettuce on the bottom of a large serving bowl, and add the thinly sliced red onion and red pepper. Add the cucumber, tomatoes, avocado, feta and sun dried tomatoes.

3. Slice the chicken and add to the salad, then sprinkle with sesame seeds and black pepper. Drizzle over some of the dressing and serve.

17. Bacon & Egg Muffin Cups with Spinach

Prep Time: 10 Minutes

Cook Time: 30 Minutes

Servings: 6

Ingredients

- 3 strips bacon
- 5 free range large eggs
- generous pinch of salt
- generous pinch of pepper
- generous pinch of garlic powder
- 1 tbsp buffalo hot sauce
- ½ cup heavy cream (110 ml)
- handful of baby spinach leaves
- ½ red bell pepper finely diced

Instructions

1. Cook the bacon, either in the oven or fry until crispy. Let cool.
2. Pre heat the oven to 180°c 360°f

3. In a jug, crack the eggs and add the salt, pepper, garlic powder, hot sauce and heavy cream Mix well.

4. Lightly grease the muffin tin with butter or oil.

5. Put in 3 or 4 baby spinach leaves into each mould, then distribute the diced bell pepper and break the bacon in to pieces and add to each mould. Pour in the egg mix

6. But the in the oven for 20-30 minutes and bake until the egg is solid.

7. Let cool slightly before serving

18. Winter Brown Rice Salad with Feta and Cranberries

Prep Time: 15 Minutes

Cook Time: 30 Minutes

Servings: 8

Ingredients

For the rice salad:

- cups wholegrain brown rice blend (16oz) (454g)
- 2 ounces arugula (55g)
- ounces walnut halves (125g)
- 7 ounces dried cranberries (200g)
- 5 ounces crumbled feta (150g)
- ounces pumpkin seeds (100g)

For the poppy seed dressing:

- ¼ cup white wine vinegar (120ml)
- 2 tablespoons granulated sugar (100g)
- 2 tablespoons poppy seeds
- pinch salt (or to taste)
- ½ teaspoon cracked black pepper
- 1 teaspoon Dijon mustard
- 3 tablespoons mayonnaise

- ½ cup extra virgin olive oil (120ml)

Instructions

For the rice salad

1. Cook the rice according to the instructions. Once cooked (do not over cook), drain and put to one side to cool to room temperature.
2. Once cool, add to a large mixing bowl. Add the rest of the ingredients and toss well.

For the poppy seed dressing

1. Whisk together the white wine and sugar.
2. Add in the poppy seeds, salt, pepper, Dijon mustard, mayonnaise and whisk together.
3. Slowly add the olive oil while whisking, until the dressing has come together.
4. When ready to serve, pour the dressing over the brown rice salad and toss.

19. Cheesy Baked Zucchini Fritters

Prep Time: 20 Minutes

Cook Time: 40 Minutes

Servings: 12

Ingredients

For the courgette fritters

- 3 medium zucchini (courgettes)
- 3 eggs
- 1.75 ounces plain flour (50g)
- ounces grated strong cheddar (100g)

For the goats cheese dip

- 4.4 ounces rindless goats cheese (125g)
- 1 tsp finely chopped chilli
- 3 tbsp sour cream
- 2 tbsp tomato passanda
- juice of ½ lemon
- 1 tsp sugar
- 1 tsp tomato puree
- 2 tsp mustard powder

Instructions

1. Top and tail the courgettes and cut into 5cm chunks. Grate the courgettes and place into a sieve. Using kitchen towel, squeeze out any excess water.

2. Crack the eggs into a large bowl and add the flour, whisk until combined. Add in the grated courgette and cheese and mix together well. Pop the mixture in the fridge and pre heat the oven to 180ºc 350F.

3. In a bowl, pop in all the ingredients for the dip and combine using a hand whisk. Put in the fridge until ready to serve.

4. Take the courgette fritter mix out of the fridge after about 15minutes. Line a large baking tray with baking paper. Place large table spoons of the mixture evenly along the baking tray, leaving gaps between, and flatten down with your fingers. Pop in the oven for around 40 minutes until golden brown. Take out of the oven and leave to cool slightly.

5. Serve the courgette fritters alongside the goats cheese dip, a few beers and some good company.

20. Green Lentil Daal

Prep Time: 10 Minutes

Cook Time: 35 Minutes

Servings: 6

Ingredients

- 4 cups green lentils 800g
- 2 tbsp olive oil
- 2 tbsp mustard seeds
- ½ tbsp turmeric
- 1 tbsp ground cumin
- ½ tbsp mild curry powder
- 2 bay leaves or 4 curry leaves if you can find them!
- 1 red onion finely diced
- 2 inches ginger minced
- 4 cloves garlic minced
- 2 red chilis minced
- 27 fl. oz coconut milk (2 cans) or cream if you want it thicker. 800ml
- 1 cup water 200 ml (more if needed)
- juice of one lime
- salt and pepper

Instructions

1. Place the lentils in a large bowl of water and set to one side. Chop the ingredients and get your spices ready!

2. Heat the oil in large pot over a medium heat. Once hot, add the mustard seeds.

3. When the mustard seeds start to pop, add in the turmeric, cumin, curry powder and bay leaves. Stir for a couple of minutes until the spices become fragrant.

4. Add in the onion, ginger, garlic and chili. Stir so that the spice coats the onions and cook for 5 minutes until the onions start to soften.

5. Drain the lentils, and add in to the pot. Add the coconut milk, lime juice and water and mix well. Pop a lid on for 15 minutes

6. After 15 minutes, take the lid off and give a good stir, at this point you can add any added vegetables that you wish. Cook the dish for another 10 or so minutes until excess liquid has cooked off

7. At this point, you could stir in some spinach or herbs - parsley and coriander work really well!

8. Serve with naan or rice

DINNER

21. (Roasted) Baked Pumpkin with Garlic and Sage

Prep Time: 15 Minutes

Cook Time: 30 Minutes

Servings: 6

Ingredients

- 1 small pumpkin (I used a pie pumpkin)
- 2 sticks salted butter (220g)
- 3 large garlic cloves
- 8 - 10 fresh sage leaves
- 1 tsp black pepper
- salt

Instructions

1. Preheat the oven to 220°c 430°f
2. Cut the pumpkin in half and scoop out the seeds. Use a good vegetable peeler to remove the skin and cut into slices around 2cm 1 inch in thickness.
3. Put a pan on a medium low heat and add the butter and slowly melt it.

4. Finely cut the garlic and sage leaves and add to the butter. Stir well and turn the heat off.

5. Line a baking tray with tin foil.

6. Put the pumpkin slices in a large bowl, and pour over the butter, add the pepper and a pinch of salt. Mix with your hands well to make sure the slices are coated.

7. Put the slices on to the lined baking tray and put in the oven.

8. Cook for 30 - 40 minutes until the pumpkin is soft and the edges are brown and crispy.

22. Thai Chicken and Rice Soup

Prep Time: 10 Minutes

Cook Time: 50 Minutes

Servings: 8

Ingredients

- 1 tablespoon oil
- 1 red chili finely chopped
- 4 garlic cloves minced
- 1 onion finely chopped
- 1 lemongrass stalk cut in half
- 2 tablespoons ginger minced
- 1 red bell pepper sliced
- 8 ounces mushrooms sliced (227g)
- 5 cups chicken stock (1.2 litres)
- 2 cans coconut milk (27 ounces 800ml)
- 2 cups brown and wild rice mix (400g 14oz)
- 2 shredded chicken breasts (400g 14 oz)
- 1 tablespoon fish sauce
- juice of one lime

To garnish (optional)

- fresh cilantro and green onion

Instructions

1. Heat the oil in a dutch oven on a medium heat on the stovetop. Add in the chili, garlic, onion, lemongrass and ginger and let it cook for 2 or 3 minutes until fragrant. Stir occasionally.
2. Add the pepper and mushrooms, give it a good stir and cook for 10 minutes. Stir occasionally so everything cooks evenly.
3. Add the stock, coconut milk, uncooked rice and shredded chicken to the pot and stir to combine.
4. Add in the fish sauce and lime juice and bring the pot to the boil.
5. Turn the heat to a medium so that the soup is simmering and place the lid and leave to cook for 30 minutes.
6. After 30 minutes, take the lid off and give the soup a stir. Turn the heat to low and cook for another 5-10 minutes to allow the soup to thicken then serve.

Prep Time: 10 Minutes

Cook Time: 35 Minutes

Servings: 4

Ingredients

- 4 cod fillets skinless and boneless (about 6-7oz 175g-200g each)
- ounces tomatoes - I used a mix of cherry and plum tomatoes, you can use whatever you have! (300g)
- 1 red pepper
- 1 teaspoon caster sugar
- 1 teaspoon salt
- 1.5 ounces parmesan (40g)
- 2 ounces pine nuts (60g)
- 1 clove of garlic
- 8 tablespoons panko breadcrumbs
- 4 tablespoons grated parmesan
- black pepper to taste

Instructions

1. Pre heat the oven to 180ºc 350ºf.

2. Slice the tomatoes in half and and put on a baking tray, cut side up. Put a bit of oil onto the red pepper and place on the baking tray. Sprinkle the salt and sugar over the cut tomatoes and pop in the oven for 20mins. Take them out and leave them to cool slightly.

3. Once cooler, remove the stalk and seeds from the pepper (you can keep the skin on) and put in a blender. Add in the tomatoes, parmesan, pine nuts and garlic. Blend until it is a smooth sauce.

4. Pre heat the oven to 180ºc 350ºf.

5. Lay the fillets of cod on a parchment lined baking tray, and put a couple of tablespoons of the red pesto over the top of each one and spread evenly over the fillets. Sprinkle on the breadcrumbs, parmesan and a little pepper to cover the sauce.

6. Bake in the oven for 15 - 20 mins until cooked through and then place them under the broiler (grill) for 5 minutes to brown the tops.

24. Chicken and Chorizo Pie

Prep Time: 20 Minutes

Cook Time: 1hr 15 Minutes

Servings: 6

Ingredients

- 1 ring of chorizo cut into chunks
- 1.3 pounds boneless skinless chicken thigh you can use breast if you prefer - cut into tasty chunks (600g)
- 3.4 ounces white wine (100ml)
- ounces chicken stock (400ml)
- 4.4 ounces shredded cheese Manchego or cheddar (125g)
- 3 tbsp cornflour or plain flour
- 1 red pepper diced
- 2 onions finely diced
- 3 cloves garlic finely diced
- 7 ounces mushrooms (200g) sliced
- 3 tbsp fresh tarragon finely chopped
- 3 tablespoons fresh parsley finely chopped
- juice of ½ a lemon
- 1 block of puff pastry

- 1 egg beaten
- flour for dusting
- Salt & pepper
- Oil for cooking

Instructions

1. Well season the chicken with salt and pepper. Pop a splash of oil into a large frying pan and cook the chorizo until crispy. Put the chorizo to one side, leaving the oil in the pan. Add the chicken chunks to the pan and brown all over. Set to one side.

2. In a separate pan, add the wine and simmer until it has reduce by about 75%, then add the chicken stock and slowly heat. To the finely grated cheese add the cornflour and make sure all the strands are covered. Add the cheese to the stock and stir occasionally until the cheese has melted - don't let this boil! Keep warm.

3. In a large saucepan, heat a splash of oil and cook the garlic, pepper and onions until soft. Stir in the mushrooms, parsley, tarragon, lemon juice and season really well with salt and pepper. Cook for 5-10 mins.

4. Add the chicken, chorizo and cheese sauce and stir well so that the sauce coats all of the ingredients. Cook for another 10mins, stirring occasionally then take off the heat.

5. Butter a large pie dish and roll out the pastry on a lightly floured surface so it is ⅛ inch thick. Cut the pastry into 1cm strips.

6. Pop the pie filling into the dish (pile it high!) and brush around the edge of the dish with the beaten egg. Place a strip of pastry vertically down the middle of the pie, then line up other strips going towards the edges, leaving a 1cm gap between the them. Then, slowly and carefully (put the wine down at this point) weave the other strips horizontally to create the lattice. Finish the pie with strips of pastry around the outside to form a frame. Once all in place brush with a coating of the beaten egg and pop in the fridge for at least 30 mins.

7. When ready to cook, pre-heat the oven to 320ºf 160ºc. Take the pie out of the fridge and pop another layer of the beaten egg on top. Bake for 40-45mins until golden brown.

Prep Time: 10 Minutes

Cook Time: 20 Minutes

Servings: 2

Ingredients

For the chicken marinade

- 1 tablespoon ground turmeric
- ¼ teaspoon black pepper
- salt
- 2 tablespoons oil (vegetable or olive oil)
- ½ teaspoon fish sauce
- 2 chicken breasts

For the sauce

- 1 can coconut milk (400ml 13.5oz)
- 3 tablespoons tomato paste
- juice of ½ a lemon
- salt and pepper

To make the dish

- 1 red onion sliced

- 1 red pepper sliced
- 2 garlic cloves thinly sliced
- 12 cherry tomatoes cut in half

Instructions

To marinade the chicken

1. Add all of the marinade ingredients to a ziplock bag along with the chicken breasts. Squeeze out any air and seal the bag. Use your hands to rub the marinade into the chicken breasts to fully coat them and place in the fridge for at least 30 minutes and up to 12 hours.

To make the sauce

2. In a large jug or bowl, combine all of the sauce ingredients and set to one side until ready to use.

To make the dish

3. Heat a pan on a medium high heat, once hot add the marinated chicken breast and cook for 3-4 minutes on each side until golden brown. Remove and set to on side.

4. In the same pan, turn the heat down slightly and add the onion, red pepper, garlic and cherry tomatoes. Cook until softened, about 5-10 minutes.

5. Add the chicken breasts back to the pan and pour the sauce in. Turn the heat to high and let it come to a simmer.

6. Give the sauce a stir, and simmer for around 5-10 minutes until the chicken is cooked through (internal temp of 165°f 75°c).

7. Sprinkle over some chopped green onion spring onion and fresh cilantro to serve.

Prep Time: 10 Minutes

Cook Time: 10 Minutes

Servings: 3

Ingredients

For the steak and marinade

- 11.5 oz flank steak
- juice of 2 lemons
- ½ teaspoon salt
- ½ teaspoon ground black pepper
- 1 tablespoon olive oil

To cook the steak

- 2 ounces salted butter preferably European style
- 2 cloves garlic peeled and slightly crushed

For the blue cheese dressing

- 1 cup sour cream (300ml)
- ⅔ cup buttermilk (250ml)
- 5 ounces blue cheese crumbled
- a couple of squeezes of fresh lemon juice

For the salad

- 1 romaine lettuce chopped
- handful of other mixed greens
- 6 radishes sliced
- ¼ large red onion sliced
- 4 mini sweet peppers sliced
- 8 to 10 cherry tomatoes halved
- 1 avocado sliced

Instructions

Marinade the steak

1. Add the steak and the marinade ingredients into a ziplock bag and remove as much air as possible. Use your hands to massage the marinade into the steak so that it's covered and place in the fridge for at least 2 hours or up to 8.

Make the blue cheese dressing

2. Add all of the ingredients to a small pan and put on a medium heat. Stir frequently until the cheese has melted and the dressing is silky smooth. Take off the the heat and let cool to room temperature. Once cooled,

transfer to a sterilized and air tight container and place in the fridge until ready to use.

Cook the steak

3. Remove the steak from the fridge 20-30 minutes before cooking it so it comes to room temperature.
4. Place the butter and garlic into a frying pan or skillet and place on a high heat.
5. Once the butter starts to bubble add the steak. Let it fry for 3-4 minutes until it has seared.
6. Flip the steak and cook of another 3-4 minutes, while spooning the butter over the top of the steak.
7. Once nicely browned, place the steak on a plate, cover with foil, and let sit for at least 10 minutes.

To build the salad

1. Chop and slice all of the salad ingredients and add to a large bowl or individual pates.
2. Once the steak has rested, slice it against the grain and place on top of the salad. Drizzle with the blue cheese dressing and serve.

Prep Time: 20 Minutes

Cook Time: 1hr 30 Minutes

Servings: 8

Ingredients

- 6 sheets of ready made filo pastry
- 1 beaten egg
- 1 ounce walnuts crushed in a mortar and pestle (25g)
- 3 beetroots
- 4 tbsp sugar
- 3 red onions finely sliced
- 4 ounces balsamic vinegar (100ml)
- 1.75 ounces red wine vinegar (50ml)
- 1.75 ounces olive oil (50ml)
- 3 eggs
- 10 ounces creme fraiche (300ml)
- 2 tbsp fresh chives finely chopped
- 7 ounces gorgonzola (200g)

Instructions

1. Pre-heat the oven to 390f 200°c.

2. Peel and top and tail the beetroots and cut them into ½ cm slices. Put on a roasting tray and sprinkle with a table spoon of caster sugar and a good pinch of salt. Place in the oven for about 20mins. Test with a knife - they should be soft with little resistance, and put to one side to cool.

3. Put the sliced onions into a saucepan and add the balsamic and red wine vinegar, along with the olive oil and 3 tablespoons of caster sugar. Put on a medium heat and stir occasionally until the liquid has evaporated. This should take about 30 minutes. Leave to one side to cool.

4. Lightly grease the dish you will be baking the tart in.

5. Take a sheet of filo and place it your dish so that the pastry comes up the sides slightly (fold the edges over if needed). Gently brush with some beaten egg and sprinkle over a small amount of the crushed walnuts. Lay another piece of filo over the top and repeat the process until you have placed on your last layer of filo. Brush well with the beaten egg and put in the oven for 10mins. Once golden brown, leave to one side to cool.

6. Turn the oven down to 355°f 180°c.

7. In a bowl, whisk together the eggs, creme fraiche and chives. Add salt and pepper to taste. Cut the gorgonzola into small cubes and stir in to the egg and cream.

8. Take the filo case, and evenly spread over the onion mixture. Place the roasted beetroot slices on top and then pour over the egg and cream mixture. Pop in the oven for 40mins, until the filling has set and the top is golden brown. Let cool before serving.

Prep Time: 20 Minutes

Cook Time: 1hr 50 Minutes

Servings: 4

Ingredients

- 2 baking potatoes
- 4 pork sausages
- ounces mushrooms finely chopped (150g)
- 2 eggs
- ounces cream cheese (100g)
- 3.5 ounces strong grated cheddar (100g)
- 4 spring onions (scallions) finely sliced
- 3 tbsp wholegrain mustard
- salt and pepper

Instructions

1. Pre-heat the oven to 430f 220°c. Rub the potatoes in a little oil, sprinkle with salt and put in the oven for 1 - 1 ½ hours until crispy on the outside. Leave to one side to cool. Keep the oven at 220°.

2. In a frying pan, cook the sausages through. Leave to one side. In the same pan, fry the mushrooms for about 10 minutes until golden brown.

3. Cut the potatoes lengthways, and scoop out the insides into a large bowl. You want to leave a thin layer of potato on the skins so they keep their shape. To the flesh, add the eggs and cream cheese, beat together well with a fork until you get a creamy consistency.

4. Cut the sausages into small chunks and add to the bowl along with the mushrooms, cheddar, onions, mustard and chilli. Give it another good mix and add a few good pinches of salt and pepper to season.

5. Spoon the mixture back into the potato skins - fill them right up! Then wrap two pieces of bacon around each potato half. Put back in the oven at 430f 220°c for around 30mins until the bacon is crispy.

Prep Time: 15 Minutes

Cook Time: 45 Minutes

Servings: 4

Ingredients

To make the caramelized onions

- 2 small red onions
- 1 tsp sugar (brown sugar is best, but whatever you have will work)
- salt and pepper (to taste)
- 1 tbsp vegetable or canola oil
- For the burger patties
- 15 ounces ground beef
- ounces panko bread crumbs
- 1 egg
- 1 teaspoon black pepper
- 1 teaspoon garlic powder
- 0.5 teaspoon salt
- 3 tablespoons black truffle oil
- 3 tablespoons runny honey

- To make the truffle mayonnaise

- 6 tablespoons mayonnaise

- 1 teaspoon black truffle oil

To build the burger

- slices of brie

- 4 burger buns (brioche or sourdough are my favorites)

- romaine lettuce

Instructions

Make the onions

1. Heat the oil in a frying pan on a medium/ high heat.

2. Slice the onions thinly and place in the pan with the sugar and a pinch of salt and pepper.

3. Stir occasionally. It will take about half an hour for the onions to cook. When they are done, put to one side.

4. While the onions are cooking, make the burgers

5. Add all of the burger ingredients to a bowl. Using your hands, mix the ingredients together. Don't over mix! Roll the mixture into a ball.

6. Cut the ball into four, and shape the patties, again, don't overwork them. Lightly cover them, and put them in the fridge for at least twenty minutes.

Make the truffle mayonnaise

1. Mix the mayo and truffle oil together. Put it in the fridge until ready to use.

Cook the burgers

2. Before cooking the burgers, take them out of the fridge and allow them to come to room temperature.
3. Heat a little oil in a frying pan on a medium to high heat, when the oil is hot, add the patties (two at a time if you have a small pan).
4. Cook one side of the patties for around 4 to 5 minutes and flip - they shouldn't be too dark when you flip them over, as you will be cooking this side again.
5. After another 5 minutes, flip again, this time the flipped side should be darker.
6. Add the caramalized onions and then the slices of brie to the top of the burgers and cover the pan with a lid to help the cheese melt. This will take about another 4 or 5 minutes.

Build your burgers

1. Toast the flat sides of your burger buns - not to toast, but so they have a little crisp to them. Spread the truffle mayo over each burger half.

2. Add some romaine lettuce on top of the burger bun and place the burger patty with the onions and cheese on top. Finish with the top of the bun.

Prep Time: 10 Minutes

Cook Time: 15 Minutes

Servings: 4

Ingredients

For the marinated chicken

- 2 chicken breast (organic and free range)
- 2 tbsp olive oil
- ½ tbsp dried oregano
- ½ tbsp dried basil
- ½ tbsp dried rosemary
- ¼ tbsp ground black pepper
- ⅛ tsp salt
- ¼ tsp garlic powder
- juice and zest of 2 lemons

For the salad

- ½ iceberg or romaine lettuce shredded
- ½ small red onion finely sliced
- 1 red pepper finely sliced
- ½ cucumber finely sliced

- 12 cherry tomatoes cut in half
- 1 avocado sliced
- to 5 ounces marinated feta cheese (100 to 150g)
- 2 sundried tomatoes finely sliced
- 1 tbsp sesame seeds
- ground black pepper
- For the salad dressing
- ¾ cup extra virgin olive oil
- ¼ cup white wine vinegar
- 1 garlic clove minced
- 1 tbsp Italian seasoning
- ¼ tsp ground black pepper
- juice and zest of ½ lemon
- ¼ tsp salt
- 1 tbsp sugar

Instructions

To marinade the chicken

1. Put all of the ingredients for the marinaded chicken (except for the chicken) into a jug and mix well.
2. Put the chicken breasts into a zip lock bag, and pour over the marinade. Close the bag and use your hands to

move the marinade around and coat the chicken. Put in the fridge for at least 30 mins - up to 2 hours for a stronger flavor.

For the salad dressing

1. Mix together all of the ingredients for the dressing and store in the fridge until ready to use.

To put it all together

2. When you are ready to cook the chicken, add a little oil to a grill pan and put on a medium high heat. Cook on both sides for around 15 to 20 minutes til cooked through. You can also use an outdoor grill.

3. While the chicken is cooking you can prep the salad. Layer the iceberg lettuce on the bottom of a large serving bowl, and add the thinly sliced red onion and red pepper. Add the cucumber, tomatoes, avocado, feta and sun dried tomatoes.

4. Slice the chicken and add to the salad, then sprinkle with sesame seeds and black pepper. Drizzle over some of the dressing and serve.

www.ingramcontent.com/pod-product-compliance
Lightning Source LLC
Chambersburg PA
CBHW050843260726
48660CB00006B/2415